INSULIN RESISTANCE DIET PLAN

Transform your Health with Delicious Recipes for Balanced Blood Sugar

Dr linda miller

Copyright Page

[insulin resistance diet plan]

Copyright © [2024] by [Dr Linda Miller]

TABLE OF CONTENT

PART 1: Introduction

Sarah, a young woman newly diagnosed with insulin resistance, felt overwhelmed. The doctor's advice was clear: diet and exercise. But how? She stumbled upon "The Insulin Resistance Cookbook," a vibrant guide with delicious recipes and clear explanations.

The book wasn't just a collection of recipes; it was a roadmap to a healthier lifestyle. Sarah learned about portion control, mindful eating, and the importance of choosing whole, unprocessed foods. She swapped sugary drinks for water and replaced white bread with whole grains.

The recipes were simple, flavorful, and adaptable. She started with a hearty lentil soup, followed by a vibrant salmon salad with avocado. Each meal felt like a celebration of healthy choices.

As Sarah diligently followed the plan, she noticed a difference. Her energy levels soared, her cravings subsided, and her weight began to stabilize. The cookbook became her trusted companion, a constant reminder that managing insulin resistance wasn't about deprivation, but about nourishing her body with love and care.

Understanding Insulin Resistance

What is Insulin Resistance?

Insulin resistance is a metabolic condition where the body's cells become less responsive to the hormone insulin, which is essential for regulating blood sugar levels. When the body detects that cells aren't responding properly to insulin, the pancreas produces more of it to help glucose enter the cells. Over time, this excessive demand on the pancreas can lead to its dysfunction, resulting in elevated blood glucose levels and potentially progressing to type 2 diabetes.

Causes and Risk Factors

Insulin resistance is often influenced by a combination of genetic and lifestyle factors. Key causes include a diet high in processed foods and sugars, lack of physical activity, obesity, and chronic stress. Certain conditions, such as polycystic ovary syndrome (PCOS) and sleep disorders like sleep apnea, can also increase the risk. Genetics play a role too; if you have a family history of type 2 diabetes, you may be more prone to developing insulin resistance.

Symptoms and Diagnosis

Insulin resistance often develops gradually and may go unnoticed until it progresses significantly. Common symptoms include fatigue, hunger, difficulty concentrating, weight gain (especially around the abdomen), and dark patches of skin (acanthosis nigricans). Diagnosing insulin resistance typically involves blood tests that measure fasting glucose, insulin levels, and an oral glucose tolerance test. Early detection is crucial to managing and reversing the condition.

The Importance of Diet in Managing Insulin Resistance

A key component of treating insulin resistance is diet. By adopting a balanced and thoughtful approach to eating, it's possible to significantly reduce insulin resistance and its associated risks. Foods that stabilize blood sugar levels, such as those with a low glycemic index, can help improve the body's response to insulin. Moreover, a well-planned diet can help with weight management, reduce inflammation, and improve overall metabolic health.

Dietary Guidelines

Focus on Low Glycemic Index (GI) Foods:

Low-glycemic foods take longer to digest and absorb, which causes blood sugar levels to rise gradually. Incorporating these foods into your diet helps in maintaining stable blood glucose levels, thereby reducing the strain on your pancreas and improving insulin sensitivity. Low-GI foods include non-starchy vegetables, most fruits, whole grains, and legumes.

Importance of Fiber and Whole Grains

Fiber, particularly soluble fiber, is essential for managing insulin resistance. It lowers blood sugar levels by slowing down digestion. Whole grains, which are rich in fiber, also have a low glycemic index and the day. It's also important to be mindful of calorie intake, as weight management is a critical component in reversing insulin resistance.

The Role of Exercise

Regular physical activity is one of the most effective ways to combat insulin resistance. Exercise helps increase the sensitivity of muscle cells to insulin, allowing them to use glucose more effectively. Both aerobic exercises, like walking or swimming, and resistance training, like weightlifting, are beneficial. Combining a balanced diet with regular exercise creates a powerful synergy that can significantly improve insulin sensitivity and overall health.

Insulin Resistance Diet Plan Overview

Goals

1. Regulate Blood Sugar: Focus on low-glycemic index foods.

. Balanced Nutrition: Include healthy fats, lean

provide sustained energy. Foods like oats, barley, brown rice, and quinoa should be staples in your diet to promote insulin sensitivity and overall metabolic health.

Incorporating Healthy Fats

Healthy fats are an important part of an insulin resistance diet. Unsaturated fats, found in foods like avocados, nuts, seeds, and olive oil, can help reduce inflammation and improve insulin sensitivity. Omega-3 fatty acids, found in fatty fish like salmon and mackerel, also play a crucial role in reducing the risk of heart disease, which is often associated with insulin resistance.

Managing Portions

Portion control is key in managing insulin resis
Eating large meals can cause spikes in bloo
levels, leading to increased insulin produc
consuming smaller, more frequent meals
help keep your blood sugar levels stable

provide sustained energy. Foods like oats, barley, brown rice, and quinoa should be staples in your diet to promote insulin sensitivity and overall metabolic health.

Incorporating Healthy Fats

Healthy fats are an important part of an insulin resistance diet. Unsaturated fats, found in foods like avocados, nuts, seeds, and olive oil, can help reduce inflammation and improve insulin sensitivity. Omega-3 fatty acids, found in fatty fish like salmon and mackerel, also play a crucial role in reducing the risk of heart disease, which is often associated with insulin resistance.

Managing Portions

Portion control is key in managing insulin resistance. Eating large meals can cause spikes in blood sugar levels, leading to increased insulin production. By consuming smaller, more frequent meals, you can help keep your blood sugar levels stable throughout the day. It's also important to be mindful of calorie intake, as weight management is a critical component in reversing insulin resistance.

The Role of Exercise

Regular physical activity is one of the most effective ways to combat insulin resistance. Exercise helps increase the sensitivity of muscle cells to insulin, allowing them to use glucose more effectively. Both aerobic exercises, like walking or swimming, and resistance training, like weightlifting, are beneficial. Combining a balanced diet with regular exercise creates a powerful synergy that can significantly improve insulin sensitivity and overall health.

Insulin Resistance Diet Plan Overview

Goals

1. Regulate Blood Sugar: Focus on low-glycemic index foods.

2. Balanced Nutrition: Include healthy fats, lean

proteins, and fiber-rich carbs.

3. Portion Control: Maintain appropriate serving sizes to avoid spikes in blood sugar.

Daily Structure:

- Breakfast: High-protein, low-carb meal to start the day.

- Snack: Fiber-rich to maintain satiety.

- Lunch: Balanced with lean protein and non-starchy vegetables.

- Snack: Healthy fats and low-glycemic fruits.

- Dinner: A mix of proteins, healthy fats, and low-GI carbohydrates.

- Snack: Light and protein-rich.

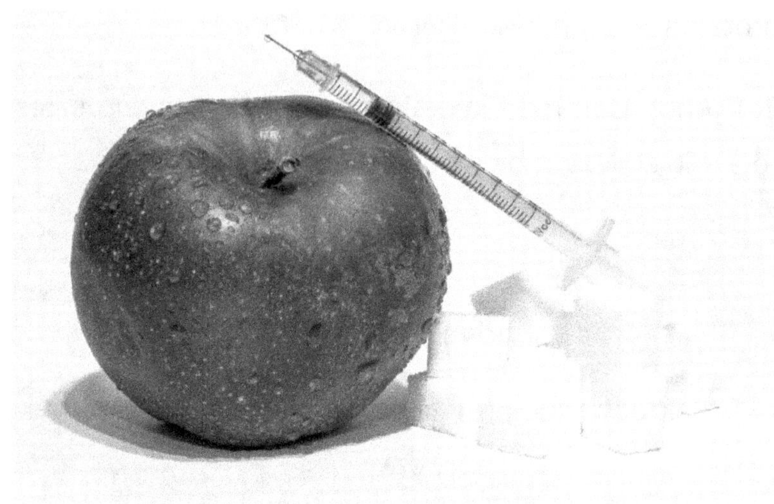

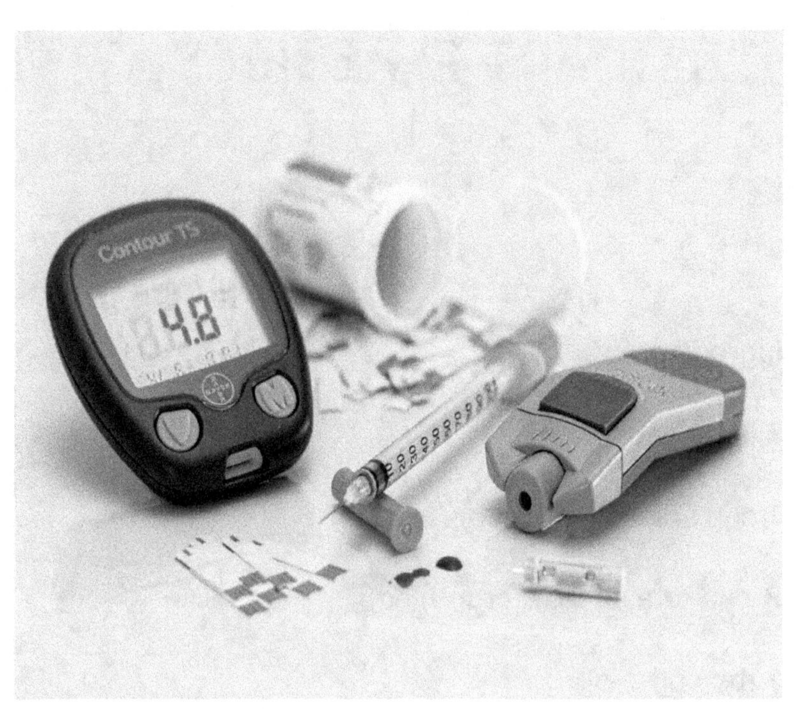

PART 2: RECIPES

Breakfast

1. Spinach and Feta Omelette

Ingredients:

3 large eggs

1 cup spinach (fresh or frozen)

¼ cup feta cheese, crumbled

1 tbsp olive oil

Salt and pepper to taste

Instructions:

1. 1. In a nonstick skillet over medium heat, warm the olive oil.

2. Add spinach and sauté until wilted, about 2 minutes.

3. In a bowl, whisk the eggs, then pour them into the skillet.

4. Cook the eggs for 2-3 minutes until they begin to set, then sprinkle feta cheese on one half.

5. Fold the omelette and cook for another 1-2 minutes until fully cooked.

6. Add salt and pepper to taste and serve.

Preparation Time: 10 minutes

Nutritional Value per Serving:

Calories: 260

Protein: 18g

Carbohydrates: 3g

Fiber: 1g

Fat: 20g

2. Chia Seed Pudding with Berries

Ingredients:

3 tbsp chia seeds

1 cup unsweetened almond milk

1 tsp vanilla extract

1 tbsp maple syrup (optional)

½ cup mixed berries (strawberries, blueberries, raspberries)

Instructions:

1. In a bowl, mix chia seeds, almond milk, vanilla extract, and maple syrup.

2. Stir well to combine, and let it sit for 5 minutes. Stir again to avoid clumping.

3. Place a lid on the bowl and chill it for a minimum of two hours or overnight.

4. Top with mixed berries before serving.

Preparation Time:

10 minutes (plus 2 hours for chilling)

Nutritional Value per Serving:

Calories: 200

Protein: 5g

Carbohydrates: 25g

Fiber: 10g

Fat: 10g

3. Greek Yogurt with Nuts and Seeds

Ingredients:

1 cup plain Greek yogurt

1 tbsp flaxseeds

1 tbsp chia seeds

2 tbsp walnuts, chopped

1 tsp honey (optional)

Instructions:

1. Place Greek yogurt in a bowl.

2. Top with flaxseeds, chia seeds, walnuts, and honey.

Preparation Time:

5 minutes

Nutritional Value per Serving:

Calories: 250

Protein: 17g

Carbohydrates: 18g

Fiber: 6g

Fat: 14g

4. Avocado Toast with Poached Egg

Ingredients:

1 slice whole-grain bread

½ avocado, mashed

1 large egg

1 tbsp olive oil

Salt, pepper, and red pepper flakes to taste

Instructions:

1. Toast the slice of whole-grain bread.

2. Spread mashed avocado on the toast.

3. In a small pot, bring water to a simmer, and poach the egg for 3-4 minutes.

4. Place the poached egg on top of the avocado toast.

5. Drizzle with olive oil and season with salt, pepper, and red pepper flakes.

Preparation Time:

10 minutes

Nutritional Value per Serving:

Calories: 300

Protein: 10g

Carbohydrates: 20g

Fiber: 7g

Fat: 22g

5. Oatmeal with Almond Butter and Flaxseeds

Ingredients:

½ cup rolled oats

1 cup unsweetened almond milk

1 tbsp almond butter

1 tbsp ground flaxseeds

1 tbsp maple syrup (optional)

Instructions:

1. In a small pot, bring almond milk to a simmer.

2. Add rolled oats and cook for 5 minutes, stirring occasionally.

3. Remove from heat and stir in almond butter, ground flaxseeds, and maple syrup.

4. Serve warm.

Preparation Time:

10 minutes

Nutritional Value per Serving:

Calories: 280

Protein: 8g

Carbohydrates: 35g

Fiber: 8g

Fat: 12g

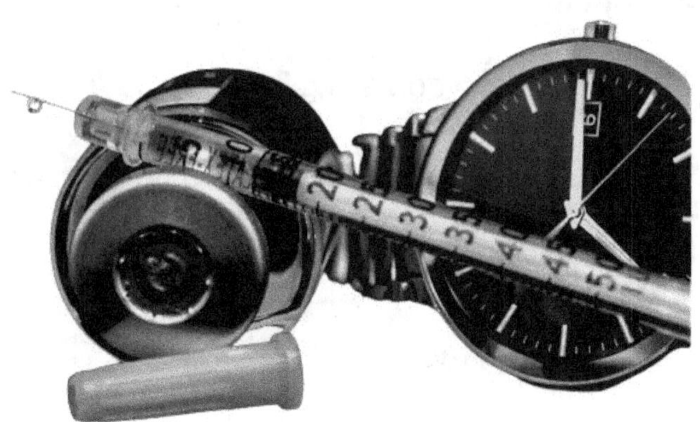

Snack

1. Greek Yogurt with Berries and Almonds

Ingredients:

1 cup plain Greek yogurt

½ cup mixed berries (strawberries, blueberries, raspberries)

2 tbsp sliced almonds

1 tsp honey (optional)

Instructions:

1. Place Greek yogurt in a bowl.

2. Add sliced almonds and mixed berries over top.

3. Drizzle with honey if desired.

Preparation Time:

5 minutes

Nutritional Value per Serving:

Calories: 200

Protein: 15g

Carbohydrates: 20g

Fiber: 5g

-Fat: 9g

2. Peanut butter-topped apple slices

Ingredients:

1 medium apple, sliced

2 tbsp natural peanut butter

Instructions:

1. Core and slice the apple.

2. Spread peanut butter on each slice or dip the slices into the peanut butter.

Preparation Time:

5 minutes

Nutritional Value per Serving:

Calories: 200

Protein: 4g

Carbohydrates: 26g

Fiber: 4g

Fat: 9g

3. Celery Sticks with Hummus

Ingredients:

 celery sticks

¼ cup hummus

Instructions:

1. Wash and cut the celery sticks into bite-sized pieces.

2. Serve with hummus for dipping.

Preparation Time:

5 minutes

Nutritional Value per Serving:

Calories: 120

Protein: 3g

Carbohydrates: 12g

Fiber: 4g

Fat: 7g

4. Hard-Boiled Eggs with Cherry Tomatoes

Ingredients:

2 large eggs

1 cup cherry tomatoes

Instructions:

1. Put the eggs in a pot and add water to cover them.

2. Bring the water to a boil, then reduce heat and simmer for 9-10 minutes.

3. Drain the eggs and let them cool before peeling.

4. Serve with cherry tomatoes.

Preparation Time:

10 minutes

Nutritional Value per Serving:

Calories: 160

Protein: 12g

Carbohydrates: 6g

Fiber: 2g

Fat: 10g

5. Cottage Cheese with Flaxseeds

Ingredients:

½ cup cottage cheese

1 tbsp ground flaxseeds

½ tsp cinnamon (optional)

Instructions:

1. Transfer the cottage cheese to a little bowl.

2. Sprinkle with ground flaxseeds and cinnamon.

Preparation Time:

3 minutes

Nutritional Value per Serving:

Calories: 120

Protein: 12g

Carbohydrates: 5g

Fiber: 2g

Fat: 6g

Lunch Recipes

1. Grilled Chicken Salad with Avocado and Quinoa

Ingredients:

4 oz grilled chicken breast

1 cup cooked quinoa

2 cups mixed greens

½ avocado, sliced

½ cucumber, sliced

1 tbsp olive oil

1 tbsp balsamic vinegar

- Salt and pepper to taste

Instructions:

1. In a large bowl, combine mixed greens, quinoa, cucumber, and avocado.

2. Top with sliced grilled chicken breast.

3. Drizzle with olive oil and balsamic vinegar, and toss to combine.

4. Season with salt and pepper, and serve.

Preparation Time:

15 minutes

Nutritional Value per Serving:

Calories: 450

Protein: 30g

Carbohydrates: 30g

Fiber: 8g

Fat: 20g

2. Turkey and Avocado Wrap

Ingredients:

1 whole-grain wrap

3 oz sliced turkey breast

½ avocado, sliced

1 cup spinach leaves

1 tbsp Dijon mustard

Instructions:

1. Spread Dijon mustard on the whole-grain wrap.

2. Layer turkey, avocado, and spinach leaves on the wrap.

3. Roll up the wrap tightly and slice in half to serve.

Preparation Time:

10 minutes

Nutritional Value per Serving:

Calories: 350

Protein: 25g

Carbohydrates: 30g

Fiber: 10g

Fat: 15g

3. Lentil and Vegetable Soup

Ingredients:

1 cup cooked lentils

2 cups vegetable broth

1 carrot, chopped

1 celery stalk, chopped

1 onion, chopped

1 garlic clove, minced

1 tbsp olive oil

Salt, pepper, and thyme to taste

Instructions:

1. In a pot, warm the olive oil over medium heat.

2. Sauté onion, garlic, carrot, and celery for 5 minutes until softened.

3. Add cooked lentils and vegetable broth, and bring

to a simmer.

4. Season with salt, pepper, and thyme.

5. Cook for 10 minutes until vegetables are tender.

Preparation Time:

20 minutes

Nutritional Value per Serving:

Calories: 250

Protein: 15g

Carbohydrates: 35g

Fiber: 12g

Fat: 6g

4. Quinoa and Black Bean Salad

Ingredients:

1 cup cooked quinoa

½ cup black beans, drained and rinsed

½ cup corn kernels

1 red bell pepper, chopped

2 tbsp cilantro, chopped

1 tbsp olive oil

1 tbsp lime juice

Salt and pepper to taste

Instructions:

1. Put cooked quinoa, black beans, corn, red bell pepper, and cilantro in a big bowl.

2. Add a lime juice and olive oil drizzle.

3. Add salt and pepper to taste, then mix to blend.

Preparation Time:

15 minutes

Nutritional Value per Serving:

Calories: 320

Protein: 10g

Carbohydrates: 50g

Fiber: 12g

Fat: 10g

5. Tuna Salad with Mixed Greens

Ingredients:

1 can (5 oz) tuna in water, drained

2 cups mixed greens

½ cucumber, sliced

1 small tomato, chopped

1 tbsp olive oil

1 tbsp lemon juice

Salt and pepper to taste

Instructions:

1. In a bowl, mix drained tuna with olive oil, lemon juice, salt, and pepper.

2. In a separate bowl, toss mixed greens, cucumber, and tomato.

3. Top the greens with the tuna mixture and serve.

Preparation Time:

10 minutes

Nutritional Value per Serving:

Calories: 200

Protein: 25g

Carbohydrates: 8g

Fiber: 3g

Fat: 8g

Dinner

1. Baked Salmon with Roasted Vegetables

Ingredients:

6 oz salmon fillet

1 cup broccoli florets

1 cup cauliflower florets

1 tbsp olive oil

1 tsp garlic powder

1 tsp lemon juice

Salt and pepper to taste

Instructions:

1. Preheat the oven to 400°F (200°C).

2. Transfer the salmon fillet to a parchment paper-lined baking sheet.

3. Drizzle with lemon juice, and season with salt, pepper, and garlic powder.

4. Toss broccoli and cauliflower with olive oil, salt, and pepper.

5. 5. Arrange the vegetables around the salmon on the baking sheet.

6. Bake for 15-18 minutes or until the salmon is cooked through and vegetables are tender.

Preparation Time:

25 minutes

Nutritional Value per Serving:

Calories: 400

Protein: 35g

Carbohydrates: 10g

Fiber: 4g

Fat: 22g

Ingredients:

1 cup tofu, cubed

1 cup broccoli florets

1 cup cooked brown rice

1 tbsp soy sauce (low sodium)

1 tbsp sesame oil

1 garlic clove, minced

1 tsp ginger, minced

1 tbsp sesame seeds (optional)

Instructions:

1. Heat sesame oil in a skillet over medium heat.

2. Add tofu and cook for 5 minutes until golden brown.

3. Add garlic, ginger, and broccoli, and stir-fry for 5 minutes.

4. Stir in soy sauce and cook for another 2 minutes.

5. Serve over cooked brown rice and sprinkle with sesame seeds.

Preparation Time:

20 minutes

Nutritional Value per Serving:

Calories: 350

Protein: 15g

Carbohydrates: 40g

 Fiber:6g

- Fat: 16g

Ingredients:

4 oz chicken breast

1 cup cauliflower rice (grated or processed cauliflower)

1 tbsp olive oil

1 garlic clove, minced

1 tbsp parsley, chopped

Salt and pepper to taste

Lemon wedge for serving

Instructions:

1. Season the chicken breast with salt and pepper.

2. Heat a grill pan over medium-high heat and cook the chicken for 5-7 minutes on each side until cooked through.

3. In a separate pan, heat olive oil over medium heat and sauté garlic until fragrant.

4. Add cauliflower rice and cook for 5 minutes until tender.

5. Stir in chopped parsley and season with salt and pepper.

6. Serve the grilled chicken over the cauliflower rice, with a lemon wedge on the side.

Preparation Time:

20 minutes

Nutritional Value per Serving:

Calories: 280

Protein: 30g

Carbohydrates: 8g

Fiber: 3g

Fat: 14g

Ingredients:

6 oz cod fillet

1 tsp olive oil

1 tsp lemon zest

1 garlic clove, minced

1 tbsp parsley, chopped

Salt and pepper to taste

1 cup asparagus spears

Instructions:

1. Preheat the oven to 375°F (190°C).

2. Transfer the fish fillet to a parchment paper-lined baking sheet.

3. Drizzle with olive oil and season with lemon zest, garlic, parsley, salt, and pepper.

4. Bake for 15-18 minutes until the fish is opaque and

flakes easily with a fork.

5. While the cod is baking, steam the asparagus for 5-7 minutes until tender.

6. Serve the baked cod with steamed asparagus.

Preparation Time:

25 minutes

Nutritional Value per Serving:

Calories: 220

Protein: 28g

Carbohydrates: 7g

Fiber: 3g

Fat: 8g

5. Turkey Meatballs with Zucchini Noodles

Ingredients:

4 oz ground turkey

1 garlic clove, minced

1 tbsp onion, minced

1 tbsp parsley, chopped

1 egg white

Salt and pepper to taste

2 medium zucchinis, spiralized into noodles

1 tbsp olive oil

1 cup marinara sauce (low sugar)

Instructions:

1. Preheat the oven to 375°F (190°C).

2. In a bowl, combine ground turkey, garlic, onion, parsley, egg white, salt, and pepper.

3. Using a baking sheet covered with parchment paper, shape the mixture into small meatballs.

4. Bake until thoroughly done, 15-20 minutes.

5. While the meatballs are baking, heat olive oil in a skillet over medium heat.

6. Add zucchini noodles and sauté for 2-3 minutes until tender.

7. Heat marinara sauce in a separate pot.

8. Serve the turkey meatballs over the zucchini noodles, topped with marinara sauce.

Preparation Time:

30 minutes

Nutritional Value per Serving:

Calories: 350

Protein: 30g

Carbohydrates: 18g

Fiber: 4g

Fat: 18g

6. Beef and Vegetable Stir-Fry

Ingredients:

4 oz lean beef strips

1 cup broccoli florets

1 carrot, sliced

1 red bell pepper, sliced

1 tbsp soy sauce (low sodium)

1 tbsp olive oil

1 garlic clove, minced

1 tsp ginger, minced

1 tsp sesame oil

1 tsp sesame seeds (optional)

Instructions:

1. Heat olive oil in a skillet over medium-high heat.

2. Add beef strips and cook for 3-4 minutes until browned. Remove from skillet and set aside.

3. In the same skillet, add garlic, ginger, broccoli, carrot, and red bell pepper. Sauté the veggies for 5 to 6 minutes, or until they are crisp-tender.

4. Return the beef to the skillet and add soy sauce and sesame oil. Stir to combine.

5. Cook for an additional 2 minutes.

6. Serve hot, sprinkled with sesame seeds if desired.

Preparation Time:

20 minutes

Nutritional Value per Serving:

Calories: 320

Protein: 28g

Carbohydrates: 15g

Fiber: 5g

Fat: 16g

7. Brussels sprouts and Baked Chicken Thighs

Ingredients:

2 bone-in, skin-on chicken thighs

1 tbsp olive oil

1 cup Brussels sprouts, halved

1 garlic clove, minced

1 tsp thyme

Salt and pepper to taste

Instructions:

1. Preheat the oven to 400°F (200°C).

2. Use thyme, salt, and pepper to season the chicken thighs.

3. In an oven-safe skillet, preheat the olive oil over medium heat.

4. Add chicken thighs, skin-side down, and cook for 5-6 minutes until the skin is golden brown.

5. Flip the chicken thighs, add Brussels sprouts and garlic to the skillet, and transfer to the oven.

6. Bake for 20-25 minutes until the chicken is cooked through and the Brussels sprouts are tender.

7. Serve hot.

Preparation Time:

30 minutes

Nutritional Value per Serving:

Calories: 400

Protein: 25g

Carbohydrates: 10g

Fiber: 4g

Fat: 28g

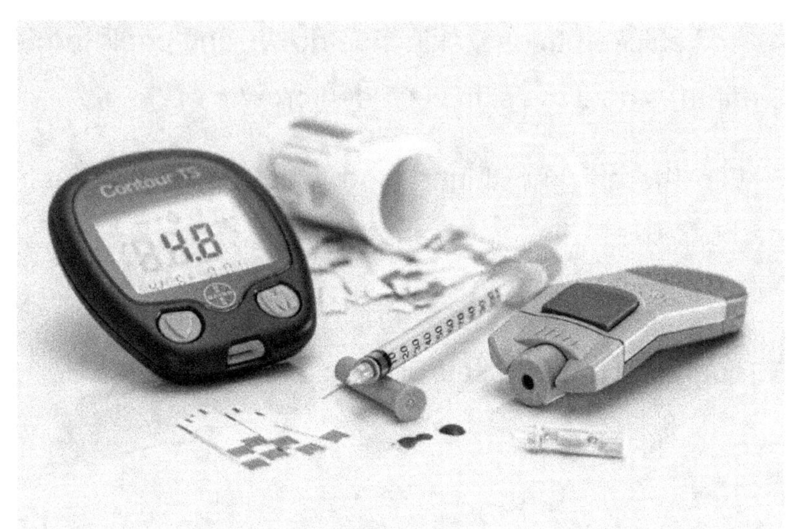

VOLUME EQUIVALENT(DRY)

U.S. STANDARD	METRIC(APPROXIMATE)
1/8 teaspoon	0.5 ml
1/4 teaspoon	1 ml
1/2 teaspoon	2 ml
1/4 teaspoon	4 ml
1 teaspoon	5 ml
1 teaspoon	15 ml
1/4 cup	59 ml
1/3 cup	118 ml
1/2 cup	156 ml
2/3 cup	177 ml
1 cup	235 ml
2 cups or 1 pint	475 ml
3 cups	700 ml
4 cups or 1 quart	1 L

www.ingramcontent.com/pod-product-compliance
Lightning Source LLC
Chambersburg PA
CBHW061313250726

48653CB00002B/917